Contents

KU-581-966

PREFACE

In 1979, the Thirty-second World Health Assembly launched the Global Strategy for health for all by the year 2000 by adopting resolution WHA32.30. In this resolution the Health Assembly endorsed the Report and Declaration of the International Conference on Primary Health Care, held in Alma-Ata, USSR, in 1978. In the same resolution, the Health Assembly invited the Member States of WHO to act individually in formulating national policies, strategies and plans of action for attaining this goal, and collectively in formulating regional and global strategies, using as a basis the guiding principles issued by WHO's Executive Board in the document entitled Formulating Strategies for Health for All by the Year 2000. *A large number of countries in all regions have since formulated national strategies, and all regions have drafted regional strategies. The Global Strategy that follows has been based on the Alma-Ata Report and Declaration and the Executive Board's guiding principles; it reflects the national and regional strategies as seen from a global perspective. It also responds to resolution 34/58 of the United Nations General Assembly concerning health as an integral part of development, which was adopted in November 1979.*

This Global Strategy for health for all by the year 2000 was adopted by the Thirty-fourth World Health Assembly in resolution WHA34.36, which reads as follows:

The Thirty-fourth World Health Assembly,

Recalling WHO's constitutional objective of the attainment by all peoples of the highest possible level of health, the Declaration of Alma-Ata, and resolutions WHA30.43, WHA32.30, and WHA33.24 concerning health for all by the year 2000 and the formulation of strategies for attaining that goal, as well as resolution 34/58 of the United Nations General Assembly concerning health as an integral part of development;

Having reviewed the Strategy submitted to it by the Executive Board in the document entitled "Global strategy for health for all by the year 2000";

Considering this Strategy to be an invaluable basis for attaining the goal of health for all by the year 2000 through the solemnly agreed, combined efforts of governments, people and WHO;

1.   ADOPTS the Global Strategy for health for all by the year 2000;

2.   PLEDGES WHO's total commitment to the fulfilment of its part in this solemn agreement for health;

3.   DECIDES that the Health Assembly will monitor the progress and evaluate the effectiveness of the Strategy at regular intervals;

4.   INVITES Member States:

(1)   to enter into this solemn agreement for health of their own volition, to formulate or strengthen, and implement, their strategies for health for all accordingly, and to monitor their progress and evaluate their effectiveness, using appropriate indicators to this end;

(2)   to enlist the involvement of people in all walks of life, including individuals, families, communities, all categories of health workers, non-governmental organizations, and other associations of people concerned;

5.   REQUESTS the Executive Board:

(1)   to prepare without delay a plan of action for the immediate implementation, monitoring and evaluation of the Strategy, and submit it, in the light of the observations of the regional committees, to the Thirty-fifth World Health Assembly;

(2)   to monitor and evaluate the Strategy at regular intervals;

(3)   to formulate the Seventh and subsequent General Programmes of Work as WHO's support to the Strategy;

6.   REQUESTS the Regional Committees:

(1)   to review their regional strategies, update them as necessary in the light of the Global Strategy, and monitor and evaluate them at regular intervals;

(2)   to review the Executive Board's draft plan of action for implementing the Strategy and submit their comments to the Board in time for it to consider them at its sixty-ninth session in January 1982;

7.   REQUESTS the Director-General:

(1)   to ensure that the Secretariat at all operational levels provides the necessary support to Member States for the implementation, monitoring and evaluation of the Strategy;

(2)   to follow up all aspects of the implementation of the Strategy on behalf of the Organization's governing bodies, and to report annually to the Executive Board on progress made and problems encountered;

(3)   to present the Strategy to the United Nations Economic and Social Council and General Assembly in 1981, and report to them subsequently at regular intervals on progress made in implementing it as well as United Nations General Assembly resolution 34/58.

Executive Summary

1. The following Executive Summary, which incorporates the main features of the Global Strategy for health for all by the year 2000,[1] is intended for the reader who would like to have a general view of the Strategy at the outset.

Background

2. In 1977 the World Health Assembly decided that the main social target of governments and of WHO should be the attainment by all the people of the world by the year 2000 of a level of health that will permit them to lead a socially and economically productive life, popularly known as "health for all by the year 2000". In 1978, an International Conference on Primary Health Care, held in Alma-Ata, USSR, stated that primary health care is the key to attaining this target.

3. In 1979 the Health Assembly launched the Global Strategy for health for all when it endorsed the Alma-Ata Report and Declaration[2] and invited Member States to act individually in formulating national strategies and collectively in formulating regional and global strategies.

What is a strategy?

4. In 1979, the Executive Board of WHO issued guiding principles for formulating strategies for health for all by the year 2000.[3] In this document, the Board described a health strategy as the broad lines of action required in all sectors to give effect to health policy. The Strategy that follows describes the broad lines of action to be undertaken at policy and operational levels, nationally and internationally, in the health sector and in other social and economic sectors, to attain health for all by the year 2000.

5. Most global plans of action resulting from international conferences have been formulated at the global level in the course of these conferences. In contrast, the Global Strategy for health for all starts with countries, and is built up through regions to the global level, where the cycle is completed by focusing on support to countries. It is not a separate "WHO strategy", but rather an expression of individual and collective national responsibility, fully supported by WHO.

6. In these circumstances is a *global* strategy a viable concept? Experience, particularly that gained from the International Conference on Primary Health Care, has shown that there is a need to issue at the global level guiding principles based on national experience, to work on these in countries, and to reinforce or

---

[1] This will be referred to throughout as "the Strategy".

[2] *Alma-Ata 1978. Primary health care*, Geneva, World Health Organization, 1978 ("Health for All" Series, No. 1).

[3] *Formulating strategies for health for all by the year 2000*, Geneva, World Health Organization, 1979 ("Health for All" Series, No. 2).

modify them until an acceptable global framework is arrived at. This framework in turn has to be broad enough to encompass the needs of all Member States and of all regions, and flexible enough to permit adaptation of national and regional strategies in such a way that they reflect national and regional variations on worldwide themes. The strength of WHO's Member States lies in this very capacity to work out global themes together and apply them in their own country after appropriate adaptation.

Bases of the
Strategy

7.   The Strategy is based on the concept of countrywide health systems based on primary health care as described in the Report of the International Conference on Primary Health Care, Alma-Ata, 1978. It relies on concerted action in the health and related socioeconomic sectors following the principles of the Alma-Ata Report. It has been drafted in accordance with the Executive Board's guiding principles on formulating strategies for health for all by the year 2000, and is a synthesis of ideas derived from national and regional strategies. The Strategy is equally valid for all countries, developing and developed alike; at the same time, it lays particular emphasis on the needs of developing countries.

Main thrusts of
the Strategy

8.   The main thrusts of the Strategy are the development of the health system infrastructure, starting with primary health care for the delivery of countrywide programmes that reach the whole population. These programmes include measures for health promotion, disease prevention, diagnosis, therapy and rehabilitation. The Strategy involves specifying measures to be taken by individuals and families in their homes, by communities, by the health service at the primary and supporting levels, and by other sectors. It also involves selecting technology that is appropriate for the country concerned in that it is scientifically sound, adaptable to various local circumstances, acceptable to those for whom it is used and to those who use it, and maintainable with resources the country can afford. Crucial to the Strategy is making sure of social control of the health infrastructure and technology through a high degree of community involvement. Also spelled out is the international action to be taken to support the above national action through information exchange, promoting research and development, technical support, training, ensuring coordination within the health sector and between the health and other sectors, and fostering and supporting the essential elements of primary health care in countries.

Promotion and
support

9.   An inseparable part of the Strategy is the action required to promote and support it. This includes strengthening the ministry of health, or analogous authority representing the whole health sector, as the focal point for the national strategy. It is necessary to ensure political commitment at the highest level nationally and internationally, as well as the support of economic development planners. Professional groups inside and outside the health sector will have to be enlisted. An appropriate managerial process for national health development will have to be developed and applied, and biomedical, behavioural and health systems research oriented to support the Strategy. Policy, technical and popular

information to ensure acceptance of and involvement in the Strategy will have to be widely disseminated.

10.　Also inseparable from the Strategy is the action required to generate and mobilize all possible resources. All human resources will have to be mobilized, not only health personnel. All types of health personnel as appropriate to the country will have to be motivated and mobilized. The best use will have to be made of available human and financial resources, and investments in health will have to be increased if necessary. The international transfer of resources from developed to developing countries will have to be rationalized and these transfers increased if necessary.

Generating and mobilizing all possible resources

11.　Intercountry cooperation is an essential feature of the Strategy, because few countries will be able to formulate and implement their strategies independently. This involves both technical and economic cooperation among countries (TCDC and ECDC), and the use of WHO's regional arrangements to facilitate such cooperation.

Intercountry cooperation

12.　To monitor progress in implementing the Strategy and to evaluate its effectiveness, suitable monitoring and evaluation processes will be set up by countries as part of their managerial process for national health development. At the international level, WHO's mechanisms will be used for reporting on progress and assessing the impact of the Strategy. Indicators will be used at the global level that are useful first of all at the national level; a list of such indicators has been prepared, based on national and regional strategies.

Monitoring and evaluation

13.　WHO will be crucial for developing and implementing the Strategy through the exercise of its constitutional role in regard to international health work; this comprises in essence the inseparable and mutually supportive functions of coordination and technical cooperation. Particular attention will be paid to the formulation of the Organization's General Programmes of Work in response to the Strategy, and to the restructuring of the Organization in the light of its functions in support of the Strategy, as decided by the Thirty-third World Health Assembly.

Role of WHO

14.　Promotion and coordination will be ensured through the fulfilment by the Health Assembly, regional committees and Executive Board of their constitutional functions, and through the follow-up of resolution 34/58 of the United Nations General Assembly concerning health as an integral part of development. WHO will use the Strategy to support the International Development Strategy for the Third Development Decade, thus contributing to the New International Economic Order. The Organization will take action to gain the support of banks, funds, and multilateral and bilateral agencies. It will also promote the Strategy through nongovernmental organizations and the use of the mass media.

15. WHO will facilitate technical cooperation among its Member States, among developing countries, among developed countries, and between developing and developed countries. The Organization will act as an international clearing-house for valid technical information. It will promote and support research and development, will act as the focal point to support the establishment and application of managerial processes for national health development and will foster manpower development, particularly through the training of trainers and support to training institutions. It will use its influence to strengthen international coordination within the health sector, and will promote intersectoral action at the international level through health development advisory councils and the establishment of bilateral and multilateral arrangements with other organizations in the United Nations system.

16. To generate and mobilize the necessary resources WHO will ensure the international mobilization of people and groups who can support the Strategy, and will foster the coordinated international transfer of resources in support of the strategies of developing countries.

17. WHO will intensify its global programmes for the essential elements of primary health care. It will ensure action at national, regional and global levels. To this end, the WHO secretariat will give top priority to the Strategy. The Director-General of WHO will exercise his full constitutional responsibilities with respect to the implementation of the Strategy. At the same time, ultimate responsibility will lie with Member States.

Preparation of plan of action

18. The Strategy will be followed by the preparation of a plan of action for its implementation, including the next steps envisaged for countries, the regional committees of WHO, the Executive Board, the World Health Assembly, and the Director-General of WHO, as well as for other related sectors, particularly within the United Nations system.

Introduction

1.   In May 1977 the Thirtieth World Health Assembly adopted resolution WHA30.43 in which it decided that the main social target of governments and of WHO in the coming decades should be the attainment by all the people of the world by the year 2000 of a level of health that will permit them to lead a socially and economically productive life. This is popularly known as "health for all by the year 2000".

2.   What does "health for all" mean? It means simply the realization of WHO's objective of "the attainment by all peoples of the highest possible level of health"; and that as a minimum *all* people in *all* countries should have at least such a level of health that they are capable of working productively and of participating actively in the social life of the community in which they live. To attain such a level of health every individual should have access to primary health care and through it to all levels of a comprehensive health system. While countries might be expected to have a similar general understanding of the meaning of health for all as outlined above, each country will interpret this meaning in the light of its social and economic characteristics, health status and morbidity patterns of its population, and state of development of its health system.

3.   In 1978 an International Conference on Primary Health Care was held in Alma-Ata, USSR. This Conference, which declared that primary health care is the key to attaining health for all, issued a Declaration, as well as 22 specific recommendations and a full report on primary health care.[1] This report emphasized that health development is essential for social and economic development, that the means for attaining them are intimately linked, and that actions to improve the health and socioeconomic situation should be regarded as mutual-

---

[1] *Alma-Ata 1978. Primary health care*, Geneva, World Health Organization, 1978 ("Health for All" Series, No. 1).

ly supportive rather than competitive. The report went on to outline the essential features of primary health care and of health systems based on it, and indicated how to organize primary health care in communities as part of a comprehensive health system. The Declaration of Alma-Ata urged all governments to formulate national policies, strategies and plans of action to launch and sustain primary health care as part of a comprehensive national health system and in coordination with other sectors. It also called for urgent and effective national and international action to develop and implement primary health care throughout the world and particularly in developing countries in a spirit of technical cooperation and in keeping with a New International Economic Order.

4.   In 1979 the Executive Board of WHO issued a document entitled *Formulating Strategies for Health for All by the Year 2000*,[1] in which it put forward guiding principles and essential issues for formulating such strategies. In the same year, the Thirty-second World Health Assembly launched the Global Strategy for health for all when it adopted resolution WHA32.30. In this resolution, the Health Assembly endorsed the Report and Declaration of Alma-Ata and invited Member States of WHO to consider the immediate use of the above-mentioned document of the Executive Board, individually as a basis for formulating national policies, strategies and plans of action, and collectively as a basis for formulating regional and global strategies.

5.   In November 1979 the United Nations General Assembly adopted resolution 34/58 concerning health as an integral part of development. In this resolution, the General Assembly endorsed the Declaration of Alma-Ata, welcomed the efforts of WHO and UNICEF to attain health for all by the year 2000, and called upon the relevant bodies of the United Nations system to coordinate with and support the efforts of WHO by appropriate actions within their

---

[1] *Formulating strategies for health for all by the year 2000*, Geneva, World Health Organization, 1979 ("Health for All" Series, No. 2).

respective spheres of competence. In connexion with the preparation of a new International Development Strategy, which was considered during the Special Session of the United Nations General Assembly in 1980, the General Assembly called for careful attention to be given to WHO's contribution, which reflects the Global Strategy for health for all.

6.   A large number of countries in all regions have now formulated national strategies, and all regions have drafted regional strategies. The Global Strategy presented in this document has been formulated in accordance with the guiding principles appearing in the Executive Board's document mentioned above. In that document, the Board described a health strategy as the broad lines of action required to give effect to health policy. The Global Strategy indicates the broad lines of action to be taken in the health sector and in related social and economic sectors, nationally and internationally, with respect to all the essential issues mentioned in the Board's document. In so doing, the Strategy makes full use of the Declaration of Alma-Ata and indicates ways by which countries can develop their health systems on the basis of primary health care as described in the Report of the Alma-Ata Conference, as well as ways by which international action can support these national endeavours. The Strategy also responds to resolution 34/58 of the United Nations General Assembly by specifying joint activities in the health and related social and economic sectors that reinforce one another and contribute to human development in general and health development in particular.

7.   Finally, the Global Strategy reflects the national and regional strategies; by their very nature, the Global Strategy cannot be a mere aggregation of them, but is rather a distillation and a synthesis of them as seen from a global perspective. It will now be possible for each region to use the Global Strategy as a basis for further refining the regional strategy, each and every region taking into account the particular needs of the countries of the region. In this way, it will be possible to arrive at national and regional variations on worldwide themes, illustrating the constitutionally unifying force of WHO as an

Organization of Member States cooperating among themselves to promote and protect the health of all peoples.

Note: The text of the Strategy is presented in the future tense; it includes such phrases as "countries will..." and "countries will cooperate...". This is a reflection of the voluntary commitment of countries to attain the goal of health for all by the year 2000 on the basis of primary health care, as urged by the Declaration of Alma-Ata. It does not imply the imposition of action on countries by a supranational body. Nor does the use of the future tense imply that it will be possible to carry out the action concerned without difficulties. Also, the use of the future tense does not necessarily imply that countries are embarking on new ventures or that a number of countries are not already carrying out the activities included in the Strategy; it implies both new initiatives and the continuation and intensification of existing ones.

I. World health and related socioeconomic problems and trends

1. Health problems and socioeconomic problems are intimately interlinked. In many countries the health and related socioeconomic situation is unsatisfactory, and future trends are not encouraging. In addition, tremendous disparities exist among countries, and these are growing; disparities also exist within countries.

2. Nearly 1000 million people are trapped in the vicious circle of poverty, malnutrition, disease and despair that saps their energy, reduces their work capacity and limits their ability to plan for the future. For the most part they live in the rural areas and urban slums of the developing countries. The depth of their deprivation can be expressed by a few statistics. Whereas the average life expectancy at birth is about 72 years in the developed countries, it is about 55 years in the developing countries; in Africa and southern Asia it is only about 50 years. Whereas only between 10 and 20 out of every 1000 infants born in the developed countries die during their first year, the infant mortality rate in most developing countries ranges from nearly 100 to more than 200 per 1000. Whereas the death rate for children between 1 and 5 years old is only about 1 per 1000 in most developed countries, it averages about 20 in many developing countries and more than 30 in Africa south of the Sahara. Of every 1000 children born into poverty in the least developed countries, 200 die within a year, another 100 die before the age of 5 years, and only 500 survive to the age of 40 years.

Survival

3. Most deaths in most developing countries result from infectious and parasitic diseases. These are closely related to prevailing social and economic conditions, and impede social and economic development. About a tenth of the life of an average person in a developing country is seriously disrupted by disease. The parasitic diseases in particular are chronic and debilitating, and they are endemic

Causes of death and disease

in most poverty-stricken areas. The common infectious diseases of childhood are still rampant in the developing countries, whereas they have been reduced to minor nuisances in the developed countries. Although these diseases can be prevented by immunization, fewer than 10% of the 80 000 000 children born each year in the developing countries are being immunized against them.

4. Diarrhoeal diseases are most widespread in the developing countries; they are transmitted by human faecal contamination of soil, food and water. Only about a third of the people in the world's least developed countries have dependable access to a safe water supply and adequate sanitary facilities.

5. Diseases transmitted by insects and other vectors are also widespread in developing countries and have a serious adverse socioeconomic influence. Malaria remains the most prevalent disease, in spite of the fact that in theory it can be prevented by the routine administration of inexpensive drugs or by insecticide spraying to kill the mosquito and its larvae. Some 850 million people live in areas where malaria has only been partially controlled, and another 350 million in areas that still lack active control measures. In tropical Africa alone, at least one million children die each year from malaria.

6. Schistosomiasis, caused by a snail-borne parasite, is endemic in some 70 countries, where an estimated 200 million people are infected. Onchocerciasis or "river blindness" causes blindness in more than 20% of the adult population in some hyperendemic regions in Africa. Development projects have increased the incidence of these diseases—of schistosomiasis owing to drainage and irrigation canals providing a habitat for the snails, and of onchocerciasis owing to the spillways of dams providing a habitat for the blackfly larvae.

7. In the developed countries, on the other hand, about half of all deaths are due to cardiovascular diseases, a fifth to cancer and a tenth to accidents. These problems are increasing in the developing countries too. Environmental health problems due to industrialization and

urbanization are assuming growing importance; these same problems could affect developing countries as they build up their industries. Chronic disease increases as people grow older. In recent years there has been a steady increase in mental disorders and in social pathology such as alcohol and drug abuse. Lung cancer as well as other chronic lung diseases due to smoking, and obesity due to overeating, are common phenomena.

8.   In contrast, in the developing countries, undernutrition afflicts hundreds of millions of people, reducing their energy and motivation, undermining their performance in school and at work, and reducing their resistance to disease. In these countries as many as a fourth of the people have a food intake below the critical minimum level. Whereas the average per capita daily energy supply in the developed countries is about 3400 kilocalories (14.23 MJ), a figure far in excess of standard requirements, it is about 2400 (10.04 MJ) for most developing countries and only 2000 (8.37 MJ) for the least developed. In addition, there are great inequalities within countries; this is catastrophic for the underprivileged in many developing countries.

Undernutrition

9.   Literacy is of major importance for health; it enables people to understand their health problems and ways of solving them, and facilitates their active involvement in community health activities. Whereas the adult literacy rate is almost 100% in industrialized countries, it is only 28% in the least developed countries, and only 13% among women in those countries. Some 900 million adults in developing countries can neither read nor write, and only 4 out of every 10 of their children complete more than three years of primary school.

Literacy

10.   The economic situation has also a direct bearing on health. While the gross national product (GNP) is far from being an ideal economic indicator, particularly in relation to health for all, since it does not reflect the degree of equity in the distribution of resources, and factors tending to increase the GNP might actually be detrimental to health, nevertheless, it is still the economic indicator in most common use. In general, with some notable exceptions, countries with a

Economic situation

high gross national product have a low infant mortality rate and a high life expectancy, the opposite being the case for countries with a low GNP. Whereas the GNP per capita ranges from only US $ 200 to US $ 1000 in most developing countries, it ranges from US $ 5000 to US $ 10 000 in most developed countries. Many of the latter, in grappling with the economic problems of inflation, balance of payments, and unemployment, are experiencing falls in their GNP and are reducing public expenditure. These problems spill over to the developing countries, with the result that their GNPs, already low by world standards, decline still further.

11.   As for the growth of the GNP per capita, the prospects for most developing countries as estimated by United Nations bodies are that they will drop between 1980 and 1985 to less than 2 % a year. The per capita income of people living in the least developed countries is likely to grow by no more than 1 % a year—an average of only US $ 2 or 3 per individual. There will even be a reduction in per capita income for the more than 140 million people in the low-income countries of Africa south of the Sahara.

Health systems

12.   To add to the difficulties, health systems are poorly organized in most countries of the world. Tremendous inequalities exist between the developed and developing countries. In the latter, approximately two-thirds of the population do not have reasonable access to any permanent form of health care. In most countries, developing and developed alike, the overwhelming proportion of resources for the delivery of health care is concentrated in the large cities. In addition, these resources are devoted to expensive, highly sophisticated technology serving a small minority of the population to the neglect of primary health care for the majority. Even in the most highly developed countries, the explosive costs of health care are making it impossible to provide the complete range of health technology to the whole population. Yet social pressures are demanding this, although it is not really necessary.

Management

13.   Deficient planning and management, including inadequate cooperation with other social and economic sectors, is another afflic-

tion of health care delivery systems in many countries. All too often, multiple delivery systems act in parallel to serve the same population group in an uncoordinated manner. This, as well as inadequate training in health management and the insufficient use of good managerial practices, all lead to inefficiency in the use of resources in these countries.

14.   In many countries health personnel are not appropriately trained for the tasks they are expected to perform, or are not provided with the equipment and supplies they require. Health manpower varies greatly from country to country and includes a wide variety of different categories of people fulfilling different functions in different societies, depending on their social and economic conditions and cultural patterns. For this reason, intercountry comparisons are very difficult. Nevertheless, to illustrate the disparities among countries, in the least developed countries one health worker of all categories, including traditional practitioners, has to serve on the average 2400 people, in the other developing countries 500 people, and in the developed countries 130 people. As for medical personnel, in the least developed countries there is one doctor for an average of 17 000 people, in the other developing countries one for 2700 people, and in the developed countries one for 520 people. The corresponding figures for nurses are one for an average of 6500 people in the least developed countries, one for 1500 people in the other developing countries, and one for 220 people in the developed countries. To highlight the extremes: in the rural areas of some least developed countries there is only one doctor to serve more than 200 000 people; whereas in the metropolitan areas of some developed countries there is one doctor for only 300 people. None of these averages reveals the extremely inequitable distribution of health personnel often found within the same country. For example, in many countries there are ten times as many people for every doctor in rural areas as there are in metropolitan areas.

Health manpower

15.   The proportion of the GNP spent on health ranges from far less than 1% in many developing countries to more than 10% in many

Health expenditure

developed countries. This implies an average of a few dollars per person per year in the developing countries as compared with several hundred dollars in most developed countries! Even if the low income countries were to increase the amounts they spend on health at the rate of 10% per annum, in the year 2000 they would still be spending only about 5% of the amount now being spent in most developed countries.

Health and related socioeconomic indicators

16. Table 1 and Fig. 1 summarize the world health and socioeconomic situation by means of a number of indicators. The disparities between different types of countries are clearly illustrated.

Table 1. Health and related socioeconomic indicators

	Least developed countries	Other developing countries	Developed countries
Number of countries	29	90	37
Total population (millions)	283	3001	1131
Infant mortality rate (per 1000 liveborn)	160	94	19
Life expectancy (years)	45	60	72
Percentage of newborn with a birth weight of 2500 g or more	70 %	83 %	93 %
Coverage by safe water supply	31 %	41 %	100 %
Adult literacy rate	28 %	55 %	98 %
GNP per capita	$ 170	$ 520	$ 6230
Per capita public expenditure on health	$ 1.7	$ 6.5	$ 244
Public expenditure on health as % of GNP	1.0 %	1.2 %	3.9 %

Note: The figures in the table are weighted averages, based on data for 1980 or for the latest available year.

Fig. 1. Health and related socioeconomic indicators

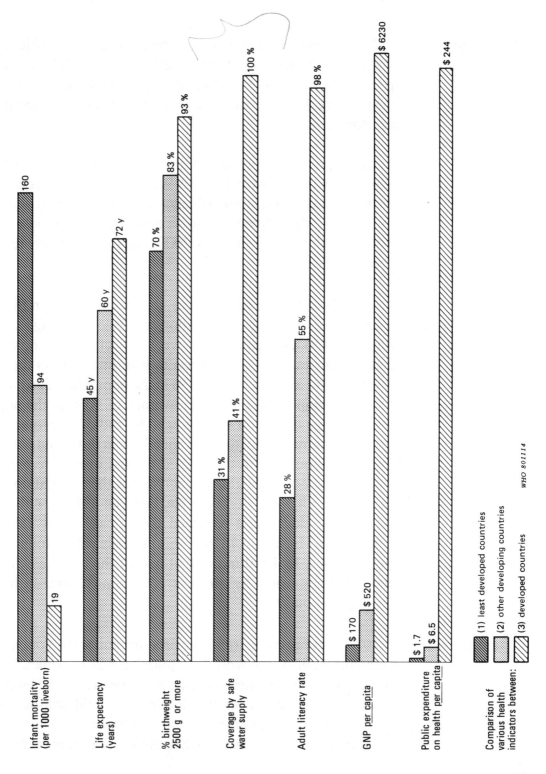

Infant mortality
(per 1000 liveborn)

Life expectancy
(years)

% birthweight
2500 g or more

Coverage by safe
water supply

Adult literacy rate

GNP per capita

Public expenditure
on health per capita

160
94
19

45 y
60 y
72 y

70 %
83 %
93 %

31 %
41 %
100 %

28 %
55 %
98 %

$ 170
$ 520
$ 6230

$ 1.7
$ 6.5
$ 244

Comparison of
various health
indicators between:

(1) least developed countries

(2) other developing countries

(3) developed countries

WHO 801114

25

Demographic
trends

17.   Trends in population growth and geographic distribution make the situation even more serious. More sick people means a greater burden on the world's economy. More healthy people would mean more human energy and therefore greater potential human development.

18.   The total population of the world increased in the 1970s at an annual rate of approximately 1.9%. If this rate of increase continues, the total world population will exceed 6000 million by the year 2000. In 1980 the developing countries accounted for almost 75% of the world population; by the year 2000, this figure is likely to increase to about 80%.

19.   Changes in age structure are also foreseen. In the developed countries, 23% of the population are below the age of 15 years, whereas 11% are aged 65 and over; projections for the year 2000 in these countries show a reduction to less than 22% in the population below 15 and an increase to 13% in the population aged 65 and over. As for developing countries, an average of 40% of the population is below the age of 15 and 4% are aged 65 and over; projections for the year 2000 show a reduction to about 34% in those under 15 and an increase to about 5% in those aged 65 and over. These percentages, however, do not highlight the increase in the population in absolute numbers at all ages. For example, between 1980 and the year 2000 the world's elderly are expected to increase from 258 million to 396 million. More than 70% of this increase will be found in developing countries. In 1980 more than half of the world's elderly lived in developed countries; by the year 2000 almost three-fifths will be in developing countries.

Urbanization

20.   If the present trend towards urbanization continues, by the year 2000 half of the world's population will be urban. Eight out of 10 people in the industrial countries will be urban residents, while the corresponding figures for the developing world will be 4 out of 10. The trend towards urbanization will result in a concentration of population in relatively few large metropolitan areas. It is estimated that by

the year 2000 out of the 15 largest metropolitan areas 12 will be in the developing countries. In spite of this trend, although the proportion of the population residing in rural areas will decline significantly, in actual numbers the rural population in the world will increase by approximately 430 million, an increase of about 500 million in the developing countries being offset by a decrease of about 70 million in the developed countries.

21. Figures 2, 3 and 4 illustrate world demographic trends until the end of the century:

Illustration of world demographic trends

22. The substantial increase in absolute numbers, and the age and geographic distribution foreseen in different groups of countries, as well as migration from rural to urban areas, all have important socioeconomic and health implications. They will influence and place

Health effects of demographic trends

Fig. 2. World population

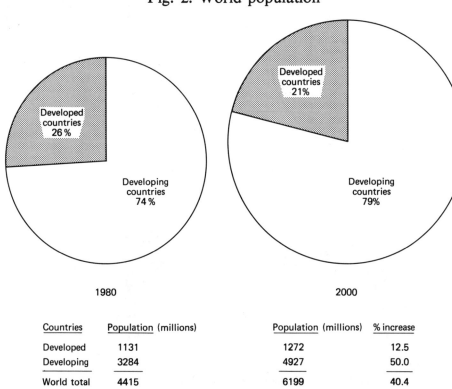

Countries	Population (millions)	Population (millions)	% increase
Developed	1131	1272	12.5
Developing	3284	4927	50.0
World total	4415	6199	40.4

additional burdens on physical and social infrastructures, increasing the dangers of unemployment and underemployment. They will affect the production and distribution of food, and they will have qualitative and quantitative implications for water, education, housing, sanitation and health care. Moreover, a change in the age structure of the population can also change the disease pattern.

Fig. 3. Age structure of the population
(Figures outside the circle show the population in millions)

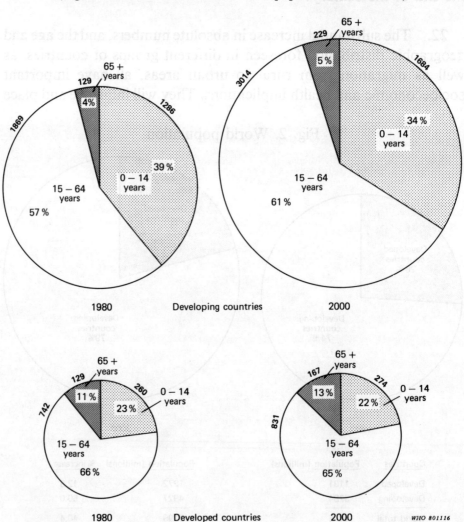

23. It is against this prospective background of complex problems and growing differentials among and within countries—regarding chances of survival; causes of death and disease; related factors such as nutritional status, water supply and sanitation, literacy, and economic situation; the organization and management of health care delivery systems; expenditures on health; and demographic trends—it is against this prospective background that the Global Strategy for health for all will have to evolve.

Prospective background for the Global Strategy

Fig. 4. Urban and rural population
(Figures outside the circle show the population in millions)

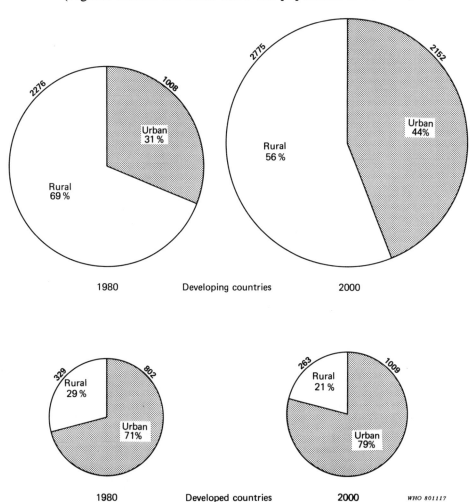

II. Health policy and related socioeconomic policy

1. The policy basis of health for all is enshrined in WHO's *Constitution*, which defines the objective of the Organization as "the attainment by all peoples of the highest possible level of health". The goal of health for all by the year 2000 embodies that objective. It emphasizes "highest possible", so that different countries will strive to improve the health of their people in keeping with their social and economic capacities. Health for all is therefore not a single, finite target; it is a process leading to progressive improvement in the health of people. Countries might be expected to have a similar general understanding of this process; however, the concept of health for all will be interpreted and adapted differently by each country in the light of its social and economic characteristics, the health status and morbidity patterns of its population, and the state of development of its health system. There is a baseline below which no individuals in any country should find themselves. The Thirtieth World Health Assembly decided in 1977 in resolution WHA30.43 that by the year 2000, *all* people in *all* countries should have a level of health that will permit them to lead a socially and economically productive life. This implies that the level of health of all people should be at least such that they are capable of working productively and of participating actively in the social life of the community in which they live. Health for all does not mean that in the year 2000 doctors and nurses will provide medical care for everybody in the world for all their existing ailments; nor does it mean that in the year 2000 nobody will be sick or disabled. It does mean that health begins at home, in schools and in factories. It is there, where people live and work, that health is made or broken. It does mean that people will use better approaches than they do now for preventing disease and alleviating unavoidable disease and disability,

and have better ways of growing up, growing old and dying gracefully. It does mean that there will be an even distribution among the population of whatever resources for health are available. It does mean that essential health care will be accessible to *all* individuals and families, in an acceptable and affordable way, and with their full involvement. And it does mean that people will realize that they themselves have the power to shape their lives and the lives of their families, free from the avoidable burden of disease, and aware that ill-health is not inevitable.

2. The International Conference on Primary Health Care, held in Alma-Ata in 1978, issued *the Declaration of Alma-Ata*, which stated that primary health care is the key to attaining health for all. It included the following definition:

"Primary health care is essential health care based on practical, scientifically sound and socially acceptable methods and technology made universally accessible to individuals and families in the community through their full participation and at a cost that the community and country can afford to maintain at every stage of their development in the spirit of self-reliance and self-determination. It forms an integral part both of the country's health system, of which it is the central function and main focus, and of the overall social and economic development of the community. It is the first level of contact of individuals, the family and community with the national health system bringing health care as close as possible to where people live and work, and constitutes the first element of a continuing health care process."

3. The Declaration of Alma-Ata also defined the essential elements of primary health care as follows:

"... education concerning prevailing health problems and the methods of preventing and controlling them: promotion of food supply and proper nutrition; an adequate supply of safe water and basic sanitation; maternal and child health care, including family planning; immunization against the major infectious diseases; prevention and control of locally endemic diseases; appropriate treatment of common diseases and injuries; and provision of essential drugs".

4. In 1979, the *World Health Assembly* launched the Global Strategy for health for all by adopting resolution WHA32.30, which endorsed the Report and Declaration of Alma-Ata and invited the Member States of WHO to act individually in formulating national

policies, strategies and plans of action for attaining this goal, and collectively in formulating regional and global strategies to support these national strategies. This combination of individual national strategies and collective international support to them is thus the backbone of the Global Strategy.

5.   Later in the same year, the United Nations General Assembly, the highest United Nations political forum, endorsed the Declaration of Alma-Ata in resolution 34/58, welcomed the efforts of WHO and UNICEF to attain health for all by the year 2000, and requested the relevant bodies of the United Nations system to coordinate with and support the efforts of WHO by appropriate action within their respective spheres of competence. Also, in connexion with the preparation of a new International Development Strategy for the Third Development Decade, it called for careful attention to be given to WHO's contribution, which reflects the Global Strategy for health for all.

6.   During the 1970s a number of international conferences were held whose outcomes were relevant to the formulation of the Global Strategy. These include the United Nations Conference on the Human Environment, the World Population Conference, the World Food Conference, the United Nations Conference on Human Settlements (HABITAT), the United Nations Water Conference, and the United Nations Conference on Technical Cooperation among Developing Countries. These two last-mentioned are particularly noteworthy. The first gave rise to the global target of safe drinking-water and adequate sanitation for all by the year 1990, and to the establishment of the International Drinking Water Supply and Sanitation Decade to reach that target; the second reinforced the existing trend towards greater cooperation among countries in health matters.

7.   Efforts to attain health for all have been supported by various groups of countries, such as the Movement of Non-Aligned Countries at its Sixth Conference of Heads of State or Government in Havana in 1979, the Organization of African Unity in connexion with the future development prospects of Africa towards the year 2000, and the Association of South-East Asian Nations.

8. Political commitment to health for all based on primary health care has also been manifested by numerous heads of state, United Nations programmes and agencies, bilateral and multilateral agencies, and international banks for development, as well as by the adoption of regional health charters in South-East Asia and Africa, to which many heads of state have made individual commitments on behalf of their governments. This should help to ensure the political and economic support required to implement the Strategy.

Fundamental policies for health for all

9. The Strategy will be based on the following fundamental policies, on which the Member States of the World Health Organization have decided through numerous resolutions in its governing bodies.

(1) Health is a fundamental human right and a worldwide social goal.

(2) The existing gross inequality in the health status of people is of common concern to all countries and must be drastically reduced. An equitable distribution of health resources, both among countries and within countries, leading to universal accessibility to primary health care and its supporting services, is therefore fundamental to the Strategy.

(3) People have the right and the duty to participate individually and collectively in the planning and implementation of their health care. Consequently, community involvement in shaping its own health and socioeconomic future, including mass involvement of women, men and youth, is a key factor in the Strategy.

(4) Governments have a responsibility for the health of their people which can be fulfilled only by the provision of adequate health and other social measures. The political commitment of the State as a whole, and not merely the ministry of health, is essential to the attainment of health for all.

(5) Countries must become self-reliant in health matters if they are to attain health for all their people. National self-reliance implies national initiative, but not necessarily national self-sufficiency.

Where health is concerned no country is self-sufficient; international solidarity is required to ensure the development and implementation of health strategies and to overcome obstacles. Such international health solidarity must respect national self-reliance.

(6) In conformity with the recognition by the United Nations General Assembly of health as an integral part of development, the human energy generated by improved health should be channelled into sustaining economic and social development, and economic and social development should be harnessed to improve the health of people. Health for all by the year 2000 cannot be achieved by the health sector alone. The coordinated efforts will be required of other social and economic sectors concerned with national and community development, in particular agriculture, animal husbandry, food, industry, education, housing, public works, and communications. Ministries of health or analogous authorities have an important role in stimulating and coordinating such coordinated action for health.

(7) Fuller and better use must be made of the world's resources to promote health and development, and thus help to promote world peace. The Strategy will therefore comply with the principles of the New International Economic Order and will contribute to its establishment and maintenance once it is established. Technical and economic cooperation among countries is crucial to the attainment of health for all since it will provide the mutual support required for the development and implementation of the Strategy. It is the best expression of international health solidarity that guarantees national self-reliance.

10.   The outline of the world health and socioeconomic situation presented in Section I illustrates the close and complex links that exist between health and socioeconomic development. The improvement of health not only results from genuine socioeconomic development as distinct from mere economic growth, it is also an essential investment in such development. In recognition of these intimate interrelationships and in compliance with the fundamental policies

Health and socioeconomic development

35

presented above, the Strategy will be based on the mutual reinforcement of health development policy and socioeconomic development policy. Full account will be taken of the extent to which the achievement of health goals will also be determined by policies that lie outside the health sector, and in particular policies aimed at ensuring universal access to the means to earn an acceptable income, whatever their nature. In many countries the conquest of poverty will be the overriding priority. According to estimates of United Nations bodies, about 800 million people throughout the world exist in conditions of absolute poverty; according to the same source, if current trends continue this figure will only be reduced to about 600 million by the year 2000. Such a situation cannot but have serious adverse repercussions on world health.

11.   But merely to increase incomes will not guarantee health. While there is a close relationship between health and income at the very lowest income levels, as incomes begin to rise health hazards associated with economic development begin to emerge. Health authorities will have to display vigilance in identifying and introducing elements that are essential for health development in national, regional, and global socioeconomic development plans. This involves making economic planners and political decision-makers aware of the health implications of alternative development strategies, identifying those aspects of development schemes which can either promote or threaten health, and ensuring that safeguards to health are incorporated into their design.

12.   Health authorities will also assure economic planners and political decision-makers that endeavours to improve health in conformity with the fundamental policies for health for all outlined above are an investment in human development. Health authorities will use the very Strategy for health for all, based on social justice and on equity in the distribution of resources for health, as an example to be followed by other sectors. They will insist on seeing evidence that investments in economic development will indeed bring about improvements in the quality of life and standard of living of people. Other sectors will be en-

couraged to take appropriate action to minimize hazards to health and to take full account of health goals as part of their own sector goals.

13. The Strategy will show the way to shaping global strategies for development in general on the basis of national strategies rather than on artificial global planning, and of cooperation rather than confrontation between developed and developing countries. It constitutes the health sector's contribution to the new International Development Strategy for the Third Development Decade, and through it to the establishment of the New International Economic Order. The paragraphs that follow illustrate some of the ways in which it will do so.

The New International Economic Order

14. The Strategy incorporates both the international and national policies for arriving at an equitable distribution of health resources and for reducing the gap between the health status of people in developing countries on the one hand and the developed countries on the other. Thus, the Strategy will help to reduce the gaps in socioeconomic status between developing and developed countries.

15. The mobilization, coordination and rationalization of the transfer of resources from bilateral and multilateral sources for the development and implementation of the national strategies of developing countries will form part of the Strategy.

16. Development of the health infrastructure will strengthen the institutional and physical infrastructures of the developing countries. Related policies of health manpower development will help to build up the critical mass of managerial, technical and scientific competence required in these countries.

17. The Strategy will comply with the principles of the New International Economic Order with respect to the transfer of technology by ensuring the provision of access to all forms of health technology, the joint search for technologies that are appropriate to the social and

economic conditions of the countries concerned, the extension of support to the developing countries to establish their self-reliance in health research and development, and collaborative research between developed and developing countries in areas of particular concern to the latter, such as tropical diseases, human reproduction, and diarrhoeal diseases.

18.   The Strategy will include the establishment of health industries in developing countries for equipment and supplies required for primary health care and the promotion of economic cooperation among these countries in this area.

19.   Sound nutritional policies will contribute to the efficient use of available food. The Strategy will also include the reaching of agreements with national and multinational food industries on standards and advertising practices.

20.   The promotion of cooperation among developing countries in formulating and implementing their strategies for health for all will strengthen technical and economic cooperation among developing countries. One example is joint bulk purchasing of essential drugs and other supplies by developing countries, which will facilitate better terms of trade in these commodities. In addition, the setting up of pharmaceutical production plant in these countries will strengthen their industrial potential.

21.   By carrying out a strategy that fulfils the above principles of the New International Economic Order, it is hoped that the health sector will act as an example to other sectors at the national and international levels.

III. Developing health systems

1. In fulfilment of the above policies, concerted efforts will be made to develop health systems of which primary health care is the central function and main focus, in conformity with the Declaration of Alma-Ata and in line with the recommendations and details concerning primary health care contained in the Report of the Alma-Ata Conference. A health system consists of interrelated components in homes, educational institutions, workplaces, communities, the health sector and other related sectors; action taken within any one component affects the action to be taken within the others. The system includes a health infrastructure which delivers a variety of health programmes and provides health care to individuals, families and communities. Such health care consists of a combination of promotive, preventive, curative and rehabilitative measures. The system is usually organized at various levels, the first of which is the point of contact between individuals and the system, where primary health care is delivered; various intermediate and central levels provide more specialized services and support as they become more central.

2. While no universal blueprint of a health system can be imposed on countries, and much remains to be done to work out the most appropriate ways of developing health systems in different national circumstances, the following principles have been defined that are applicable to all health systems based on primary health care:

(1) The system should encompass the entire population on a basis of equality and responsibility.

(2) It should include components from the health sector and from other sectors whose interrelated actions contribute to health.

(3) Primary health care, consisting of at least the essential elements included in the Declaration of Alma-Ata, should be

delivered at the first point of contact between individuals and the health system.

(4) The other levels of the health system should support the first contact level of primary health care to permit it to provide these essential elements on a continuing basis.

(5) At intermediate levels more complex problems should be dealt with, more skilled and specialized care as well as logistic support should be provided, and more highly trained staff should provide continuing training to primary health care workers, as well as guidance to communities and community health workers on practical problems arising in connexion with all aspects of primary health care.

(6) The central level should coordinate all parts of the system, and provide planning and management expertise, highly specialized care, teaching for specialized staff, the expertise of such institutions as central laboratories, and central logistic and financial support.

Building up the health system

3. Countries will review their health systems with the aim of reshaping them as necessary to conform to the above characteristics. This will imply the establishment of a well-coordinated infrastructure, starting with family and community care, and continuing with intermediate and central support and referral levels. This infrastructure will deliver well-defined health programmes that use appropriate technology and that cover the whole population, progressively if necessary.

4. Countries with well-developed infrastructures but ill-defined programmes will take measures to formulate countrywide programmes with clear objectives for delivery by the infrastructure. Countries with well-defined programmes but weak infrastructures will concentrate on strengthening their infrastructure to deliver those programmes to the total population.

5.   Some countries will concentrate initially on delivering a limited number of programmes to the whole population; others will provide a wider range of programmes to selected geographical areas or population groups, such as those in greatest need, progressively extending the number of these areas and groups; yet others will provide a complete range of health programmes to the total population, progressively improving quality. Countries concentrating on a limited number of programmes at the outset, such as malaria control, immunization, or diarrhoeal disease control, will deliver them through the general health infrastructure, thus strengthening it and acting as a spearhead for the progressive delivery of a wider range of primary health care activities through it.

6.   To develop such health systems countries will take into account the following.

(1) Action to be taken in the health sector will be identified, planned and coordinated.

(2) Action to be taken in other sectors will be identified, and the responsible authorities approached with a view to implementation.

(3) Ways will be devised of involving people and communities in decisions concerning the health system and in taking responsibility for self-care as well as family and community care.

(4) Central planning will aim at enabling communities of different types and sizes to work out their own primary health care activities.

(5) A supportive referral system will be devised and put into effect, particular attention being paid initially to the first referral level.

(6) A logistic system will be organized and operated for the whole country.

(7) Health manpower will be planned, trained and deployed in response to specific needs of people as an integral part of the health infrastructure.

(8) Appropriate health care facilities will be planned for, designed, constructed and equipped so that they are readily available, accessible and acceptable to all the population.

(9) Health technology will be selected that is scientifically sound, adaptable to various local circumstances, acceptable to those for whom it is used and to those who use it, and maintainable with resources the country can afford.

Coordination within the health sector

7. To achieve coordination within the health sector countries will pay attention to the following:

(1) collaboration between the various health services and institutions, following agreement on allocation of responsibilities in order to make the most efficient use of resources. These may include services and institutions belonging to government, social security, the private sector, nongovernmental and voluntary organizations active in the health sector, for example Red Cross or Red Crescent societies and the like, and women's and youth organizations;

(2) collaboration between the various levels of the health system following agreement on the distribution of functions and resources;

(3) collaboration within and among the various categories of health workers following agreement on the division of labour.

Intersectoral action

8. To foster intersectoral action, countries will devise ways of ensuring adequate cooperation between ministries of health or analogous authorities[1] and other ministries concerned. The role of the ministry of health will include spearheading and coordinating action. The following possibilities will be explored in particular:

(1) the establishment of multisectoral national health councils comprising personalities representing a wide range of interests in

---

[1] In the text that follows, whenever "ministry of health" is mentioned it includes an equivalent authority in some countries; whatever the title of the authority, the essential feature is that it should represent the whole health sector.

the fields of health and political, economic and social affairs, as well as the population at large, to explore jointly policy questions affecting health and socioeconomic development; including both the positive and negative effects on health of measures aimed at economic growth;

(2) the establishment of interministerial committees, or the use of existing interministerial committees for social affairs, in which the health representatives will take initiatives to promote the action in other sectors that the implementation of the strategy requires;

(3) the establishment of arrangements between ministries of health and other ministries and sectors concerned in relation to such specific fields as nutrition, water, housing, education, communications, the protection of the environment, the production and import of drugs and equipment, and use of the mass media. Since such multisectoral action is an integral part of the primary health care approach, it is described in greater detail under "Essential elements of primary health care" in paragraph 26 below;

(4) the delegation of responsibility and authority to communities to organize their own primary health care or selected elements of it, as well as to intermediate levels of the health system to provide support to primary health care; and the use of this process as an example to encourage administrative reforms in other sectors with a view to facilitating intersectoral coordination at the different administrative levels.

9. Ministries of health or analogous authorities will ensure the subdivision of the country into different types and sizes of communities in which primary health care will be organized, taking account of administrative boundaries to facilitate intersectoral collaboration. Consideration will be given to helping these communities to organize themselves, and to the correct delegation to them of responsibility, authority, and appropriate budgets. The ministry of health will provide guidelines and practical support as necessary to those communities that will organize their own primary health care.

Organizing primary health care in communities

Referral system

10. The functions of the mechanisms and institutions in the health and related sectors will be reviewed, particularly at the first referral level, and staff will be motivated and retrained as necessary to provide support and guidance to communities and community health workers.

11. A system of referral of patients and problems will be developed so that the first referral level is not overloaded with problems that could be dealt with by primary health care in the community, and so that patients and problems are referred back to those who sent them, accompanied by information on action taken and guidance for further action.

12. Ministries of health will review transport and communication facilities together with local authorities and representatives of the other ministries concerned, to permit the referral system to function efficiently.

Logistic system

13. Ministries of health will review their logistic system to ensure regular and timely distribution of supplies and equipment, as well as the availability of transport and its maintenance, starting with facilities in communities and working centrally through intermediate and central levels.

Health manpower

14. Ministries of health, in collaboration with other ministries and educational bodies concerned, will take steps at the highest government level to introduce the policy of educating and training health manpower to perform functions that are highly relevant to the country's priority health problems, in contrast to accepted practice in many countries. In fulfilment of this policy they will review the functions of health personnel throughout the health system, and will take the necessary measures to ensure their reorientation as necessary.

15. Ministries of health, together with other ministries concerned such as ministries of labour and education, will plan health manpower in specific response to the needs of the health system, with a view to

placing at the disposal of the system the right kind of manpower in the right numbers at the right time in the right place.

16. Ministries of health and other ministries and educational bodies concerned, such as ministries of education, will review training in the light of projections for the number, types and quality of the different categories of health worker required. Such training will take account of the role of health workers in supporting individuals and families to provide self-care. They will make all efforts to introduce the necessary reforms in faculties of medicine, health sciences and other relevant training institutions so that in addition to their technical training health personnel will become imbued with the philosophy of health development as defined in the Declaration and Report of Alma-Ata and in this Strategy. In view of their scarcity, particular emphasis will be given to the training of adequate numbers of "health generalists"—that is, people who can generate schemes for such health development, and plan, programme, budget, implement, monitor, and evaluate them; who can bring together to these ends the specialized knowledge of all the other disciplines involved in the health, political, social, and economic sciences; and who can marshal, master, and summarize the information required for all these activities.

17. Ministries of health and other ministries concerned, for example, for education, culture, labour, finance, and public administration, will take steps to ensure that health workers are socially motivated and provided with the necessary incentives to serve communities.

18. Ministries of health, together with ministries of public works in some countries, will review the distribution of existing health care facilities and will work out and continually update national master plans of requirements for health centres and dispensaries and for first-referral hospitals. Accessibility to those most in need will be the foundation of the master plans.

Health care facilities

19. Ministries of health will review the functions, staffing, planning, design, equipment, organization, and management of health centres and first-referral hospitals, in order to prepare them for their wider function in support of primary health care. Before investing in buildings, the cost of running them will be considered.

Health technology

20. A systematic assessment will be made of the health technology[1] being considered for use in each priority programme, aimed at applying technology that is appropriate for the country or part of the country concerned. This will include measures for health promotion, disease prevention, diagnosis, therapy, and rehabilitation. Decisions will have to be taken whether to apply these measures one by one or concurrently. The process of determining health technology will also entail specifying for each programme what measures should be taken by individuals and families in their home and what by communities, whether by individual or community behaviour or by specific technical measures. Finally, the measures to be taken by the health service at primary, secondary and tertiary levels, as well as those to be taken by other sectors, will be specified.

21. To arrive at appropriate technologies, ministries of health will involve other governmental departments concerned, such as ministries of science and education, as well as research and academic institutions, industry, and nongovernmental organizations, both in the health sector and in related sectors. They will also consult widely with communities, particularly with respect to the acceptability of the measures being proposed, to local adaptations such as rural or urban variants, and to the proper selection of local methods.

Health systems research

22. In the course of selecting appropriate measures, countries will identify the need for research to generate new technologies. They will

---

[1] "Technology" is used in the sense ascribed to it in the Alma-Ata report on primary health care—namely, "an association of methods, techniques and equipment... together with the people using them"—*Alma-Ata 1978. Primary health care*, Geneva, World Health Organization, 1978, p. 59 ("Health for All" Series, No. 1).

also apply health systems research to arrive at the best ways of incorporating technology in the measures to be taken through primary health care and the referral levels of the health system. In addition, health systems research will be used to arrive at the best ways of organizing the health system infrastructure, starting with primary health care at the first level of contact, continuing through subsequent referral levels, and testing mechanisms for intersectoral action and community involvement.

23.   Ministries of health will consider alternative ways of providing the essential elements of primary health care. Having identified for each priority programme the activities to be carried out by the people themselves, by communities, by the health service, and by other sectors, they will consider aggregating the activities to be expected from each of these categories for the sum total of all programmes. This will permit them to identify the support action required for each of these categories. For example, people will have to be supported to administer self-care, to treat common diseases and injuries, or to administer prophylactic drugs for certain endemic diseases. Efforts to change people's life-style could have a significant impact on the nutritional status of people and that of their children, on the proper use of water and sanitary facilities, and on the prevention and control of certain communicable and noncommunicable diseases.

Essential elements of primary health care

24.   In this way too it will be possible to identify the support required by communities to organize and control their own primary health care, and to take the necessary measures to influence the environment, including the psychosocial environment, with a view to preventing and controlling a wide variety of communicable diseases, other diseases such as cardiovascular diseases, cancer, and mental disorders, and such phenomena as alcohol and drug abuse.

25.   In the same way it will be possible to identify what has to be undertaken by the health system infrastructure for the totality of programmes in such diverse fields as the application of technology;

the provision of information; training; guidance and health education; clinical care; and the distribution of drugs and supplies.

26.   Ministries of health will approach other sectors with a view to motivating them to take action in specific fields. In some countries, ministries of planning, finance and agriculture will be approached, with a view to reaching a proper balance between food crops and cash crops. In many countries, the agricultural and the housing and public works sectors will be approached with respect to the provision of safe drinking-water and sanitation. Planning and development ministries will be approached to ensure that proper attention is given to health aspects of development schemes, such as the prevention of certain parasitic diseases. The educational and cultural sectors will be asked to participate in wide-ranging health educational activities in communities, schools, and other educational, training and cultural institutions. Those responsible for public works and communications will be requested to facilitate the provision of primary health care, through improved communications, particularly for dispersed populations. Access to the mass media will be facilitated through ministries of information and the like. The industrial sector will be made aware of the measures required to protect the environment from pollution and to prevent occupational diseases. The industrial sector will also be requested, as the need arises, to consider the possibility of establishing industries for essential foods and drugs. The sector of trade and commerce will be requested to consider ways of controlling the import and export of goods destined for human use that could have adverse effects on health.

Social control

27.   When the health system infrastructure and the programmes it has to deliver are specified in the above way, countries will be in a better position to deal in a practical way with the social control of the whole health system in a manner that is consonant with their political, cultural and administrative traditions. A clear national policy may be needed, and even appropriate legislative and budgetary measures, to ensure that individuals and communities can participate actively in deciding on health policy and in guiding the planning, management

and control of the health infrastructure and the programmes it delivers. Existing mechanisms may be used, or new ones may have to be created, to make it possible for people to express their views on their community's or country's health system, to take decisions concerning the scope of individual and community involvement in ensuring certain elements of primary health care in the health and related sectors, to control primary health care in the community in which they live, and to participate actively in the control of the other levels of the health system. To fulfil such responsibilities people have to be well informed; to inform them will be an important function of health personnel, who form part of the community and country in which they live and work.

28. Countries will define targets both for the development of the health system infrastructure and for programmes to be delivered by the infrastructure. This will involve setting intermediate date limits for the completion of certain activities and for the attainment of certain objectives. While such targets will by their very nature be specific to each country, the global targets presented in paragraph 37 below give an indication of the kind of target countries may consider. **Targets**

29. International action to support national action for developing health systems will concentrate on the strengthening of national health infrastructures and on the promotion of the health science and technology required to facilitate the selection by countries of technologies that are appropriate to their circumstances. The following are further details of this international action. **International action**

30. Information on national experiences will be exchanged among countries, particularly on the following issues: Information exchange

> (1) national health systems based on primary health care and how they are organized;

> (2) the development of health infrastructures based on primary health care;

(3) the organization of primary health care in communities;

(4) developments in health technology, the technologies selected by countries, and methods of selecting technology;

(5) the allocation of responsibilities for health-related activities to people, communities, the health service and other sectors;

(6) community involvement in and social control of health systems.

Research and development

31. International action in the area of research and development on health systems will take the following shape:

(1) international coordination of research to identify and generate appropriate health technology for the essential elements of primary health care;

(2) promotion and development of health systems research, including support to such research in countries, strengthening of national research institutions, intercountry collaboration, and the development of suitable research methods;

(3) research and development on specific issues of growing concern, such as self-care and the influence of life-style on health.

Technical support

32. International support of a technical nature will include the following:

(1) preparation and wide dissemination of guiding principles and related learning material on such issues as the organization of primary health care by communities; referral systems; logistic systems; and the planning, design, contruction, equipment, and management of health facilities;

(2) development of methods for assessing health technologies;

(3) technical cooperation with individual countries on request for the development of their health system.

33. International support to training for the development of health systems will include: Training

(1) training of trainers;

(2) establishing or reshaping as necessary relevant training institutions, including public health schools in developing and developed countries alike.

34. International support to coordination within the health sector will concentrate on: Promoting coordination within the health sector

(1) coordination of the fields of action of the World Health Organization and other international organizations interested in different aspects of health, for example, the human environment and social security;

(2) promotion of the mutual acceptance of different categories of health worker, and of the rationalization of the division of labour among them, through international professional bodies, and in particular nongovernmental organizations;

(3) promotion of agreement on the respective fields of endeavours of international nongovernmental organizations and voluntary bodies working in the health field.

35. Intersectoral action at the international level, will be promoted in the following ways: Promoting intersectoral action

(1) the establishment of regional health development advisory councils comprising personalities representing a wide range of interests in the fields of health and political, economic and social

affairs, to explore jointly policy questions affecting health and socioeconomic development in their region;

(2) the establishment of bilateral and multilateral arrangements between the World Health Organization and other bodies of the United Nations system on such specific issues as:
- community organization
- intersectoral health systems research
- provision of essential drugs, vaccines and cold-chain equipment to low-income developing countries
- drug and vaccine production
- inclusion of health promotive and protective components in economic development projects
- food and nutritional policies and food supplements
- inclusion of health literacy in literacy programmes
- facilitation of access to the international mass media
- protection of the human environment
- coordinated support to the International Drinking Water Supply and Sanitation Decade;

(3) the establishment of joint activities between nongovernmental organizations in the health and other sectors on priority intersectoral issues relevant to the Strategy.

Essential elements of primary health care

36.   In addition to the above support, much of which relates to the essential components of primary health care, international activity will be intensified on a global scale to foster and support the essential elements of primary health care in countries. This will include programmes to develop appropriate health technologies through scientific research, and to foster their application through national health infrastructures in the most efficient way. Particular attention will be paid to the needs of high-risk groups, such as mothers and children, workers at special risk at their place of work, and the elderly; as well as to areas hitherto neglected on an international scale, such as clinical, laboratory and radiological technology, and ensuring the provision of essential drugs to low-income developing countries.

37.   The following illustrate the kind of targets that countries will   Global targets
consider, taking into account their socioeconomic and health
situations, and that will be aimed at globally for the year 2000:

(1) All people in every country will have at least ready access to essential health care and to first-level referral facilities.

(2) All people will be actively involved in caring for themselves and their families as far as they can and in community action for health.

(3) Communities throughout the world will share with governments responsibility for the health care of their members.

(4) All governments will have assumed overall responsibility for the health of their people.

(5) Safe drinking-water and sanitation will be available to all people.

(6) All people will be adequately nourished.

(7) All children will be immunized against the major infectious diseases of childhood.

(8) Communicable diseases in the developing countries will be of no greater public health significance in the year 2000 than they are in developed countries in the year 1980.

(9) All possible ways will be applied to prevent and control noncommunicable diseases and promote mental health through influencing life-styles and controlling the physical and psychosocial environment.

(10) Essential drugs will be available to all.

IV. Promoting and supporting health system development

1. To ensure and facilitate the implementation of the policies on which the Strategy is based as outlined above, intensive efforts will be made to ensure the commitment of political decision-makers and the support of economic planners, as well as to win over the health and related professions. An adequate managerial process will be established to facilitate the implementation of the Strategy by the national health system. Health research will be reviewed and reoriented as necessary so that it gives priority to problems whose solution is required to implement the Strategy. Information, too, will be used as an operational arm to support the aims of the Strategy and facilitate its implementation.

2. The successful pursuit of the Strategy *in countries* will depend on one authority being responsible for it on behalf of the government. The first reform to be considered in many countries will therefore be to strengthen the status of the ministry of health or analogous authority so that it becomes the directing and coordinating authority on national health work. This does not necessarily imply direct administration of all health facilities, since most health systems by their very definition will include elements that are not administratively subordinate to the ministry of health; it does imply the responsibility for channelling activities into the national strategy for health for all and coordinating them on behalf of the government, both within the health sector, no matter what the executing agency or institution, as well as within other sectors through the appropriate channels. In some countries, this responsibility will devolve on the health sector as a whole, including health services provided by social security and industries as well as ministries of health, the sector being presided over by the minister of health.

Ensuring political commitment

3.   Ministries of health, relying on the collective commitment of the Member States of WHO to the Strategy, will take initiatives to ensure the commitment of their governments as a whole to its implementation within countries. In addition, on behalf of the government, they will make efforts to ensure the support of public figures and bodies as appropriate, such as political parties, religious and civic leaders, trade unions, and influential nongovernmental organizations. Popular support will be mobilized by involving individuals and families in their own health care and by involving them collectively in technical, supportive and financial community action for primary health care.

4.   Ministries of health will propose to their governments appropriate mechanisms for ensuring the action required in all relevant social and economic sectors, such as interministerial committees or multisectoral national health councils. They will deploy all means for ensuring the redistribution of resources for health so that they become progressively equitable for all segments of the population throughout the country. To introduce the necessary health reforms, in some countries enabling legislation will be promulgated—for example, to define the rights and obligations of people concerning their health, as well as those of various categories of health workers and institutions; to protect people from environmental hazards; and to permit communities to develop and manage their health and related social programmes and services. Care will be taken to avoid protracted deliberations on legislation as a substitute for action, and to ensure that people understand the nature of the legislation and approve of it.

5.   *In the international arena* use will be made of the World Health Assembly and the WHO regional committees to provide constant political support through declarations and approaches to political leaders, the United Nations system and the mass media. The formulation of health charters will be considered by those WHO regions that have not already done so, and the ratification of such charters by heads of state will be solicited. Intensive action will be taken within the United Nations system to gain the support of heads of state for the national and international strategies for health for all. The United

Nations General Assembly and the Economic and Social Council will be kept informed at suitable intervals of progress towards implementing General Assembly resolution 34/58 on health as an integral part of development, and attaining the goal of health for all. The governing bodies of the United Nations specialized agencies will be approached through the executive heads of these agencies to take action to support the Strategy in their specific fields of endeavour.

6.   Similar approaches will be made to subregional, regional and global geopolitical groupings through influential "friends of health for all" among representatives of their member countries. These geopolitical groupings will be encouraged to include in their platforms, and as an integral part of their activities, those parts of the Strategy that are relevant to them. Influential international nongovernmental organizations will also be approached to include in their activities those parts of the Strategy that fall within their fields of competence. Important developments in national health legislation in support of strategies for health for all will be brought to the attention of other countries which could possibly benefit from this information.

7.   *Ministries of health* will seize all opportunities of gaining the support of economic planners and institutions by convincing them that health is essential for development in that it contributes to production and by refuting the contention that the pursuit of health consists merely in the consumption of scarce resources for marginally useful medical care that has no impact on the health of the people. Ministries of health will also display vigilance, employing specialized personnel if necessary, in order to ensure that health needs and protective measures are made integral parts of development projects, taking account of cost-effectiveness—for example in irrigation schemes, dams, and industrial development projects in developing and developed countries alike.

Ensuring economic support

8.   *At the international level* constant efforts will be made to influence bilateral and multilateral agencies to channel resources into support for the Strategy in such a way that these resources will have a

multiplier effect in countries. Systematic measures will be taken to convince banks, funds, and multilateral and bilateral agencies to adopt firm policies of providing grants and loans for the Strategy, in recognition of its contribution to human development. Information will be gathered and widely disseminated to illustrate the benefits that can accrue from the incorporation of health protective measures in development projects as well as the adverse effects of ignoring these measures. This information will be presented in particular to regional economic commissions, to influence them to take account of the health implications of large-scale development schemes.

Winning over professional groups

9. Community involvement in developing and carrying out the national strategy for health for all also implies the involvement of people having a technical function in society bearing on health. Particular efforts will be made to ensure the support of these people who, if properly motivated, can have a powerful influence on policy-makers and the general public alike; if they are not mobilized, they can constitute a serious obstacle.

10. To secure the support of the health professions, *ministries of health* will consider ways of involving them in the practice of primary health care and in providing support and guidance to communities and community health workers. To this end they will approach the professional organizations of medical doctors, nurses, and other health professions, providing them with information, and holding dialogues with them, and impressing upon them their social responsibilities. They will also consider ways of providing tangible incentives.

11. To gain a longer-term influence, health authorities will provide incentives to public health schools, and to medical, nursing and other health-science schools, to include in their educational programmes the philosophy of health for all, the principles of primary health care, and the essentials of the managerial process for national health development, and to provide appropriate practical training in

these areas. In a similar manner, efforts will be made to involve technical workers in other sectors having a bearing on health.

12. *At the international level*, all technical nongovernmental organizations whose activities could contribute to the acceptance and promotion of health for all through primary health care will be provided with information concerning the health for all movement. They will be requested to incorporate in their programmes activities aimed at influencing their members to become deeply involved in this movement in their own countries. Such activities might consist of general progress reports, the review of specific technical issues from the perspective of the needs of countries to implement their strategies, the pursuit of research that is relevant to health for all, and the retraining of their members.

13. United Nations specialized agencies will be approached with requests to include in their programmes action relevant to the Strategy, whether to support national action by the sector concerned, or to engage the support of people in various social and economic disciplines, particularly through their nongovernmental organizations. In this way, attempts will be made to set in motion action by other United Nations bodies in support of the Strategy in such fields as socioeconomic planning and management, education, agriculture, and industrial development.

14. To permit them to develop and implement their strategies, *countries* that have not already done so will establish a permanent, systematic, managerial process for health development. Whatever the precise nature of the process, it will lead to the definition of clearly stated objectives as part of the national strategy and, wherever possible, specific targets. It will facilitate the preferential allocation of health resources for the implementation of the Strategy, and will indicate the main lines of action to be taken in the health and other sectors to implement it. It will specify the detailed measures required to build up or strengthen the health system based on primary health care

Establishing a managerial process

for the delivery of countrywide programmes. The managerial process will also specify the action to be taken so that detailed programmes become operational as integral parts of the health system, as well as the day-to-day management of programmes and the services and institutions delivering them. Finally, it will specify the process of evaluation to be applied with a view to improving effectiveness and increasing efficiency, leading to modification or updating of the Strategy as necessary. Health manpower planning and management will be an inseparable feature of the process. For all the above, the support of relevant and sensitive information will be organized as an integral part of the health system.

15. Ministries of health will establish permanent mechanisms to develop and apply their managerial process and to provide adequate training to all those who need it. These may include mechanisms in ministries themselves, as well as networks of individuals and institutions in the health and other sectors, including academic institutions, to share the managerial research, development and training efforts required for health development.

16. *International support* of both a material and technical nature will be provided to countries for the development of their managerial process and mechanisms.

17. Material support will be provided through the mobilization of human and financial resources for the establishment or strengthening of national mechanisms for developing, training the people required, and applying the managerial process, including the organization of the related information. Intercountry collaboration between these national mechanisms will be fostered.

18. Technical support will include the preparation and wide dissemination of guiding principles for the managerial process, based on national experience, that can be adapted by countries to their needs,

together with related training material. Technical cooperation with individual countries will also be ensured to help them develop, apply and train people in their managerial process. Priority will be given to the training of trainers and other senior public health officials; this will take place mainly in national health development institutions, particularly through the process of learning by doing.

19.   Research is often considered a luxury of the affluent and yet its successful pursuit and the application of its findings are often the source of affluence. *Governments* will review the scope and content of their activities in the field of biomedical, behavioural and health systems research, with a view to focusing them on problems requiring solution as part of their strategies for health for all. The identification of such problems is one of the many concerns of the managerial process for national health development. The ultimate aim will be to reach national self-reliance in health research, but governments will first identify those research activities which they can carry out using national resources, those for which international collaboration is required, and those for which it is better to rely on the efforts of countries endowed with greater resources for health research.

Reorienting research

20.   Attention will be given to the allocation of resources to relevant health research, to the training of young scientists and the related question of career structures for health research workers, to the balance between work in health research and in health service, and to the wide dissemination of research results to different audiences so that they can be speedily applied.

21.   Consideration will be given to establishing or strengthening health research councils to facilitate the coordination of health research activities within the country, to increasing the interest of medical research councils in the broad problems of health, or to creating health research sections in general scientific research councils.

22.   Mechanisms for bringing together researchers and planners, such as national health development networks, will be used to ensure that research designs meet the requirements of decision-makers and that results are actually used.

23.   *International support* to national health research will concentrate on identifying priorities for international collaborative research, coordinating the pursuit of such research in countries, providing technical support to strengthen national health research capability through training, particularly of young scientists, and by temporary secondment of experienced investigators, and mobilizing financial resources for research in less developed countries.

24.   Quite apart from progress reports on international collaborative research, research results that could be usefully applied will be disseminated widely to countries as soon as they are available; appropriate mechanisms will be developed to this end.

25.   Most of the international support to research relating to the Strategy will be generated and coordinated by WHO's regional and global advisory committees on medical research and its special research programmes.

Information

26.   Information will be used as a permanent operational arm of national and international strategies to mobilize political, financial, managerial, technical, and popular support. *Ministries of health* will assume a highly active role in disseminating the kind of information that is likely to influence various target audiences. Thus, statements on the aims and potential socioeconomic benefits of the Strategy, as well as progress reports on its implementation, will be submitted to political, economic and social leaders and to government circles concerned.

27. Information concerning the validity of various health technologies and problems encountered in their application, and methods of designing and managing health systems, will be supplied on a continuing basis to health workers of different kinds.

28. The above types of information will be popularized and disseminated to the general public through the mass media, the educational and cultural sectors, and through primary health care itself.

29. *International support* for the above will take the form of providing the world with an objective account of what is really valuable for health development and of those health problems for which there is as yet no suitable answer. This account will include the dissemination to countries of information on the global aims and potential socioeconomic benefits of the Strategy, as well as progress reports on its implementation. Similar material will be addressed to the world's political and socioeconomic leaders in appropriate international forums, such as the United Nations General Assembly and the Economic and Social Council, geopolitical groupings, and international political and socioeconomic institutes and the like.

30. Validated information on all technical and managerial issues concerning health for all through primary health care will be generated through international collaboration, and widely disseminated.

31. Popular material reflecting the political, socioeconomic, managerial, and technical information referred to above will be prepared in such a way that it can be adapted by countries to their needs. Entry points will be vigorously sought for the dissemination of this popular material at the international level, including the mass media, the film industry, nongovernmental organizations, international social and religious groups, women's groups, youth groups and the like.

V. Generating and mobilizing resources

1.   To carry out the Strategy throughout the world will mean generating and mobilizing all possible resources. Two types of resource are involved, namely, human resources and financial and material resources.

2.   The Strategy involves mobilizing all human resources, and not only health personnel. Realizing that the best way to mobilize people is to involve them, *ministries of health* will explore appropriate ways of involving people in deciding on the health system required and the health technology they find acceptable, and in delivering part of the national health programme through self-care and family care and involvement in community action for health.

Development of human resources

3.   The following are some of the measures that will be considered to promote community involvement:

(1) delegation of responsibility, authority and resources to establish primary health care in the community in a way that is linked to the real-life situation of the people in the community;

(2) creation of community health councils, composed of representatives of a cross-section of the people in the community, to develop and control primary health care;

(3) fostering individual responsibility for self-care and family care, adopting a healthy life-style, and applying the principles of good nutrition and hygiene;

(4) delegation of responsibility and resources to communities to carry out agreed components of health programmes, such as insecticide spraying against malaria and ensuring adequate nutrition for underprivileged children;

(5) developing mechanisms for people to participate at the national level in decision-making on the country's health system and health technology through accepted social and political channels;

(6) ensuring people's representation in national or intermediate-level health councils;

(7) election of members of the public to the governing bodies of health institutions.

4. Ministries of health will launch countrywide health educational activities through health personnel and the mass media and in educational institutions of all types, with the aim of enlightening the whole population on the prevailing health problems in their country and community and on the most appropriate methods of preventing and controlling them.

5. At the same time, full attention will be given to the reorientation and retraining as necessary of existing health workers, including measures to enable them to assume an active role in community health education. Consideration will also be given to the development of new categories of health workers, to the involvement and reorientation as necessary of traditional medical practitioners and birth attendants where applicable, and to the use of voluntary health workers.

6. In addition to the orientation and training of health workers, other people with community responsibility, such as civic and religious leaders, teachers, community workers, social workers, and magistrates, will be provided with information on the national health strategy and the part they could play in supporting it.

7. Voluntary organizations will be given full encouragement to participate in health-promoting activities, first aid and other health care following agreed courses of action and distribution of responsibilities.

8. *At the international level* the following action be taken:

(1) Information will be collated and used internationally regarding people and groups throughout the world who could provide individual or group support to countries on various aspects of their strategies.

(2) Specific tasks will be identified for international nongovernmental and voluntary organizations, and a systematic drive will be made to enlist their commitment to carrying them out.

(3) UNESCO will be requested to use information relating to health in its worldwide literacy programme, with a view to providing an elementary understanding of nutritional and health needs and of how to prevent or control common health problems.

(4) The developing and developed countries concerned will be brought together to agree on practical measures for preventing the brain-drain of health personnel.

9. Just as the successful implementation of the Strategy will mean mobilizing all possible human resources, it will also depend on mobilizing all possible financial and material resources. This implies first of all making the most efficient use of existing resources both within and among countries. At the same time, additional resources will undoubtedly have to be generated.

Financial and material resources

10. In this context *ministries of health* will:

(1) review the distribution of their health budget and in particular allocations to primary health care and intermediate and central levels, to urban and rural areas, and to specific underserved groups;

(2) reallocate existing resources as necessary—or, if this proves impossible, at least allocate any additional resources—for the provision of primary health care, particularly for underserved population groups;

(3) include an analysis of needs in terms of costs and materials in all consideration of health technology and of the establishment and maintenance of the health infrastructure;

(4) consider the benefit of various health programmes in relation to the cost, as well as the effectiveness of different technologies and different ways of organizing the health system in relation to the cost;

(5) estimate the order of magnitude of the total financial needs to implement the national strategy up to the year 2000;

(6) attempt to secure additional national funds for the strategy if necessary and if they are convinced that they can prove that they have made the best possible use of existing funds;

(7) consider alternative ways of financing the health system, including the possible use of social security funds;

(8) identify activities that might attract external grants or loans;

(9) in developing countries take action so that their governments request such grants and loans from external banks, funds and multilateral and bilateral agencies;

(10) in developed countries, take action to influence the agencies concerned to provide such grants and loans;

(11) present to their government a master plan for the use of all financial and material resources, including government direct and indirect financing; social security and health insurance schemes; local community solutions in terms of energy, labour, materials and cash; individual payments for service; and the use of external loans and grants.

11. *International action* will consist of the following:

(1) exchange of information on alternative ways of financing health systems;

(2) the estimation of the order of magnitude of financial and material needs for the Strategy;

(3) promotion of, development of methodology for, and support to cost-benefit studies on various aspects of the Strategy, such as programmes for safe water and adequate sanitation, immunization, and nutrition, and cost-effectiveness studies on various ways of organizing health systems based on primary health care;

(4) resource transfers from developed countries to developing countries that are ready to devote substantial additional resources to health, and review of the nature and size of such transfers with the aim of satisfying the needs of the Strategy;

(5) strengthening the capacities of developing countries to prepare proposals for possible funding by their governments and from external sources;

(6) the establishment of regional mechanisms to identify needs and facilitate national mobilization of funds as well as transfers between countries;

(7) the establishment of a global Health for All Resources Group where representatives of developed and developing countries, bilateral and multilateral agencies, and certain United Nations organizations as well as nongovernmental organizations and foundations, can get together under the auspices of WHO to rationalize the transfer of resources and seek ways of generating additional funds as necessary.

12.   About US $ 20 000 million are being spent annually as public   Cost estimates
expenditure on health in the developing countries (calculation based on the figures in Table 1 in Section I above). Little is known about private expenditure on health in these countries, including payment in cash or in kind to traditional medical practitioners and birth attendants. There are as yet no accurate estimates of the cost of attaining health for all by the people of these countries by the year 2000,

although a number of tentative analyses have been made. For example, according to certain preliminary rough estimates an annual addition of about US $ 10 per head for health in developing countries could have far-reaching effects. To support developing countries in finding these additional funds, it would be necessary to transfer to them annually about US $ 2 per head for about 400 million people; about US $ 1 per head for about 800 million people; about US $ 0.5 per head for a further 800 million people to provide them with the information and technical support they require. This leads to the need for a total annual transfer of about US $ 2000 million. In addition, the transfer of about US $ 3000 million a year is required for safe water and adequate sanitation, and this should be shared by the relevant sectors throughout the world both inside and outside the United Nations system. These rough estimates will be progressively refined as further information becomes available.

13.   Out of the above grand total of about US $ 5000 million required in international transfers for health, about US $ 2000 million are already being transferred. Of these, about US $ 1200 million come from bilateral sources and about US $ 700 million from non-governmental organizations. In addition, about US $ 1000 million are provided in the form of bank loans and United Nations activities related to health, but these are not strictly speaking transfers.

14.   The total expenditure on health in the developed countries has been estimated as being about twice the public expenditure, thus amounting to an annual average over the next two decades of about US $ 600 000 million (calculation based on Table 1 and Fig. 2 in Section I above). The Strategy could in all probability be implemented by most developed countries at no extra cost through the reshaping of their health systems as necessary and the judicious reallocation of existing resources accordingly.

VI. Intercountry cooperation

1. It is clear from the scope and complexity of the national strategies outlined above that few countries will be able to implement them independently. This underscores the need for intercountry cooperation, which is the form most international support will take.

2. Ministries of health will therefore approach their governments to ensure commitment not only to implement their own strategy but to cooperate fully with other countries to implement the Global Strategy.

3. Such cooperation is of particular importance to developing countries (TCDC), as is economic cooperation among them (ECDC).

Technical and economic cooperation among developing countries

4. Developing countries will consider participating in TCDC/ECDC in cooperative activities and joint ventures such as, for example, the exchange of information and experience on all aspects of their strategies, training, collaborative research, use of one another's experts, joint programmes for the control of certain diseases, production, procurement and distribution of essential drugs and other essential medical equipment and supplies, development and construction of health infrastructural facilities, and the development and application of low-cost technology for water supply and waste disposal.

5. Developed countries, too, will consider intensifying cooperative activities, for example, in such areas as the assessment of clinical, laboratory and radiological technology and of the usefulness of selective health screening for early detection of disease, research on prevalent noncommunicable diseases and mental health, control of environmental hazards, including the long-term health effects of chemicals in the environment, prevention and control of alcohol and drug abuse, accident prevention, and the care of the elderly.

Technical cooperation among developed countries

6.   The lessons learned from activities such as the above will be made available to all countries, developed and developing alike.

Cooperation among developed and developing countries

7.   Cooperation among developed and the developing countries will be mutually beneficial in implementing national strategies and will be indispensable for implementing the Global Strategy. In keeping with the principles of the New International Economic Order, new forms of trilateral and multilateral cooperation for health development will take place, involving both developed and developing countries and the World Health Organization.

WHO's regional arrangements

8.   WHO's regional arrangments will be fully used by countries to facilitate cooperation among them. The regional strategies for health for all, which contribute to the Global Strategy, will be adapted as necessary so that they reflect global considerations and continue to deal with the specific applications required by countries in the region in the light of their socioeconomic and health situations.

VII. Monitoring and evaluation

1. *Governments* will want to know if they are making progress with the implementation of their strategies, and whether these strategies are having the desired effect in improving the health status of the people. To this end they will consider introducing at the earliest stage a process of monitoring and evaluation that is appropriate to their needs as part of their managerial process for national health development. Whatever the precise nature of the process, it should include monitoring progress in carrying out the measures decided upon, the efficiency with which these measures are being carried out, and the assessment of their effectiveness and impact on the health and socioeconomic development of the people.

National monitoring and evaluation process

2. Monitoring of implementation and evaluation of effectiveness and impact normally take place at two levels—the policy level and the managerial and technical levels—but the two have to be interlinked. At the policy level countries will wish to know if the health status of the population is improving and if revisions of the health policy and strategy are required. At the managerial and technical levels, those concerned will wish to know if relevant programmes are being formulated and if corresponding services and activities for implementing them are being adequately designed. They will also wish to know if programmes are being efficiently implemented through suitably operated health and related social and economic services.

3. As part of their process of evaluation countries will select indicators that are appropriate to their social, economic and health situation. In doing so, they will be highly selective so that the use of indicators becomes manageable and meaningful. Since socioeconomic and health situations are evolutionary, the selection of indicators will be correspondingly evolutionary. Health policy and socioeconomic indicators, health status and quality of life indicators, and indicators

National indicators

of the delivery of health care, will be taken into account. In all cases, the selection of indicators will be heavily influenced by the feasibility of collecting the information required.

4. *International support* will be made available to countries to help them decide on their health evaluation process and to select indicators, firstly through the issue of specific publications on these matters.

Regional and global monitoring and evaluation

5. Monitoring and evaluation of the Strategy will also take place at regional and global levels. In this way countries will cooperate in assessing progress being made collectively in regions and globally towards attaining the goal of health for all. Monitoring and evaluation at these levels will be based in information received from countries. This cooperative process will provide all countries with information on the prevailing health and related socioeconomic situation and will facilitate taking decisions on any needed modifications to international health policy and to the Global Strategy.

Global indicators

6. A short list of indicators will be used for global monitoring and evaluation of the Strategy. This implies the commitment of countries, individually as well as collectively in regional groupings, to use at least these indicators and provide the necessary information on them. It is stressed that these constitute a minimal list so that all countries may be in a position to use them. Many countries will wish to use additional indicators in keeping with their needs and capacities. To this end they may find useful the WHO publication entitled *Development of Indicators for Monitoring Progress Towards Health for All by the Year 2000*.[1] Since average global values of indicators have little meaning, monitoring and evaluation at the global level will rely on indicators expressed in terms of the number of countries, as follows:

---

[1] *Development of indicators for monitoring progress towards health for all by the year 2000*, Geneva, World Health Organization, 1981 ("Health for All" Series, No. 4).

The number of countries in which:

(1) *Health for all has received endorsement as policy at the highest official level*, e.g., in the form of a declaration of commitment by the head of state; allocation of adequate resources equitably distributed; a high degree of community involvement; and the establishment of a suitable organizational framework and managerial process for national health development.

(2) *Mechanisms for involving people in the implementation of strategies have been formed or strengthened, and are actually functioning*, i.e., active and effective mechanisms exist for people to express demands and needs; representatives of political parties and organized groups such as trade unions, women's organizations, farmers' or other occupational groups are participating actively; and decision-making on health matters is adequately decentralized to the various administrative levels.

(3) *At least 5% of the gross national product is spent on health.*

(4) *A reasonable percentage of the national health expenditure is devoted to local health care*, i.e., first-level contact, including community health care, health centre care, dispensary care and the like, excluding hospitals. The percentage considered "reasonable" will be arrived at through country studies.

(5) *Resources are equitably distributed*, in that the per capita expenditure as well as the staff and facilities devoted to primary health care are similar for various population groups or geographical areas, such as urban and rural areas.

(6) *The number of developing countries with well-defined strategies for health for all, accompanied by explicit resource allocations, whose needs for external resources are receiving sustained support from more affluent countries.*

(7) *Primary health care is available to the whole population, with at least the following:*

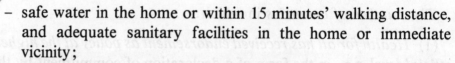

- safe water in the home or within 15 minutes' walking distance, and adequate sanitary facilities in the home or immediate vicinity;
- immunization against diphtheria, tetanus, whooping-cough, measles, poliomyelitis, and tuberculosis;
- local health care, including availability of at least 20 essential drugs, within one hour's walk or travel;
- trained personnel for attending pregnancy and childbirth, and caring for children up to at least 1 year of age.

(8) *The nutritional status of children is adequate, in that:*
- at least 90% of newborn infants have a birth weight of at least 2500 g;
- at least 90% of children have a weight for age that corresponds to the reference values given in Annex 1 to *Development of Indicators for Monitoring Progress Towards Health for All by the Year 2000*, cited above.

(9) *The infant mortality rate for all identifiable subgroups is below 50 per 1000 live-births.*

(10) *Life expectancy at birth is over 60 years.*

(11) *The adult literacy rate for both men and women exceeds 70%.*

(12) *The gross national product per head exceeds US $ 500.*

Reporting on progress and assessing impact

7.   In view of WHO's role as the directing and coordinating authority on international health work, in accordance with Article 2 of its Constitution, and the obligation of Member States to submit reports to WHO in accordance with Articles 61 and 62 of its Constitution, countries will use the mechanisms of WHO for reporting on progress and assessing the impact of the Strategy. Reports on progress will be reviewed by regional committees every two years. The regional reviews will be followed by global reviews by WHO's Executive Board and World Health Assembly. A report on progress

made towards attaining health for all by the year 2000 will be published biennially beginning in 1983. Every six years regional followed by
global assessments will be made to evaluate the effectiveness of the
Strategy.

VIII. The role of WHO

1.   As stated in Section VI above, most international support will take the form of intercountry cooperation. It is part of WHO's constitutional role as the directing and coordinating authority on international health work to foster and support this cooperation, since the Organization's international health work comprises in essence the inseparable and mutually supportive functions of coordination and technical cooperation. Such technical cooperation has become fundamentally different from traditional technical assistance. The specific functions of WHO with respect to the Strategy will also be determined by such Health Assembly resolutions as WHA23.59, on the important functions of the Organization; WHA33.17, on the study of WHO's structures in the light of its functions; and WHA32.24, together with resolution 34/58 of the United Nations General Assembly, concerning coordination of activities with other organizations of the United Nations system to attain health for all. WHO's role will thus include coordinating all aspects of the Strategy and cooperating with Member States as well as facilitating cooperation among them regarding the Strategy. In particular, WHO will place itself at the disposal of its Member States to facilitate technical cooperation and economic cooperation among developing countries.

2.   To perform its international health work in the above spirit, the Organization's General Programmes of Work will be formulated in such a way as to promote, coordinate and support efforts by the countries of the world individually and collectively to implement successfully the Strategy for health for all. They will consist of priority issues for WHO action, and the broad lines for such action, in the health sector as well as in other sectors concerned as far as WHO can have an influence on them.

WHO's General Programmes of Work

3.   To this end, the Organization will continue to be restructured at national, regional and global levels to permit its regional committees, Executive Board and World Health Assembly, as well as its

WHO's structures in the light of its functions

Secretariat, to carry out the responsibilities devolving on them in accordance with resolution WHA33.17 on the study of WHO's structures in the light of its functions.

Promotion and coordination

4. The development of the Strategy was set in motion by the World Health Assembly; the Health Assembly will have overall responsibility for approving it, monitoring its implementation, and evaluating it. The regional strategies, of which the Global Strategy is a synthesis, and which are themselves a synthesis of national strategies, have been agreed upon by the regional committees; these committees will be responsible for monitoring the implementation of the regional strategies, evaluating them, and updating them as necessary.

5. The Health Assembly and regional committees will be active in promoting the Strategy at the highest political levels in countries, in geopolitical groupings of countries, in the United Nations system, in international nongovernmental and voluntary organizations, and in the mass media. The Health Assembly will be particularly active in following up resolution 34/58 of the United Nations General Assembly on health as an integral part of development.

6. WHO will play a leading role in ensuring economic support for the Strategy at the international level by convincing international banks, funds, multilateral and bilateral agencies to adopt firm policies of providing grants and loans for the Strategy.

7. WHO will also assume the leading role in international attempts at winning over professional groups to support the Strategy through nongovernmental organizations and the United Nations specialized agencies.

8. WHO will use information as an operational arm for mobilizing the widespread support for the Strategy of people throughout the world in all walks of life.

9. On behalf of its Member States, the Organization will cooperate with other intergovernmental agencies in supporting the new International Development Strategy through the Global Strategy for Health for All, and in this way will contribute to the New International Economic Order.

10. WHO will strengthen its capacity to facilitate TCDC by reorienting its programme activities accordingly and by establishing any necessary mechanisms as part of its restructuring. This will encompass cooperation among developing countries, among developed countries, and among developed and developing countries. The Organization will create mechanisms for ensuring timely and appropriate exchanges of information among countries interested in the possibility of technical cooperation among themselves. It will also participate in joint efforts with other international organizations inside and outside the United Nations system to supply countries with information conducive to TCDC and to support them technically and managerially as required to ensure the success of such cooperation. Whereas the financing of TCDC activities will be mainly the responsibility of the countries themselves, WHO will assist countries in obtaining external financial support for it as necessary.

TCDC

11. WHO will act as an international clearing-house for validating and disseminating technical information on:

Technical information

(1) the development of health infrastructures and related managerial processes and health systems research;

(2) the delivery of primary health care with the support of the rest of the health system;

(3) the selection, adjustment and generation of appropriate health technologies;

(4) the social control of health systems and health science and technology;

(5) intersectoral action for health.

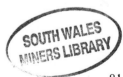

Research and development

12.   WHO will support countries in strengthening their capacities for organizing and conducting biomedical, behavioural and health systems research related to the implementation of their strategies. The Organization's regional and global advisory committees on medical research and its special research programmes will be the main instruments for promoting and coordinating the international research and development required for the successful implementation of the Strategy.

Management

13.   WHO will act as the world focal point to help countries develop their managerial process for national health development and apply it to implement their strategies. The Organization's activities will include:

(1)   the preparation and wide dissemination of guiding principles and related training material for the managerial process;

(2)   cooperation with individual countries on request in developing, applying and providing appropriate training in their managerial process, particularly the training of trainers and other senior public health officials;

(3)   international mobilization of resources to strengthen national institutional infrastructures engaged in developing, applying and providing training in the managerial process.

Training

14.   In support of the Strategy WHO will concentrate on the following with respect to training:

(1)   training of trainers;

(2)   establishing or reshaping training institutions in developing countries;

(3)   cooperating with developed countries with a view to reshaping their public health schools and other relevant training institutions as necessary.

15.   WHO will assume the responsibility of strengthening coordination within the health sector at the international level with a view to strengthening it at the national level. To this end, the Organization will make concrete proposals for coordinated action to selected international, governmental, nongovernmental and voluntary organizations.

Coordination within the health sector

16.   WHO will promote intersectoral action at the international level, with a view to supporting it at the national level, in the following ways:

Promoting intersectoral action

(1) the establishment of international, intersectoral health development advisory councils;

(2) the establishment of bilateral and multilateral arrangements between the World Health Organization and other parts of the United Nations system, including the following:

- United Nations Children's Fund (UNICEF)—community organization; training in the formulation of health strategies; intersectoral health systems research; provision of essential drugs, vaccines and cold-chain equipment to low-income developing countries; all activities relating in particular to the health of children;
- World Bank, Regional Development Banks, and United Nations Development Programme (UNDP)—inclusion of health promotive and protective components in economic development projects;
- Regional Economic Commissions—inclusion of health promotive and protective components in regional economic development projects;
- the United Nations, UNICEF, UNDP, the United Nations Environment Programme (UNEP), the International Labour Organisation (ILO), the Food and Agriculture Organization of the United Nations (FAO), the United Nations Educational, Scientific and Cultural Organization (UNESCO), and the World Bank—coordinated support to the International Drinking Water Supply and Sanitation Decade;

– FAO and World Food Programme (WFP)—food and nutritional policies and food supplements;

– UNESCO—inclusion of information on health in literacy programmes, and facilitation of access to the international mass media;

– United Nations Fund for Population Activities (UNFPA)—family planning and related aspects of maternal and child health;

– UNEP—protection of the human environment;

– United Nations Industrial Development Organization (UNIDO) —drug and vaccine production;

(3) the establishment of joint activities between nongovernmental organizations in the health and other sectors on priority intersectoral issues relevant to the Strategy.

Generating and mobilizing resources

17. WHO will use its own regular budget and programme activities as a launching pad to promote the generation and mobilization of resources for health within countries and the transfer of resources for health from developed to developing countries.

18. To mobilize *human resources* WHO will:

(1) engage in technical cooperation with its Member States and foster such cooperation among them, to ensure the maximum mobilization and deployment of people for health;

(2) organize the collation and international use of information regarding people and groups who can provide support to the Strategy;

(3) lead the drive to enlist the involvement of international nongovernmental and voluntary organizations;

(4) promote dialogues between developing and developed countries to prevent the brain-drain of health personnel.

19. To mobilize *financial resources* the Organization will:

(1) ensure the exchange of information on alternative ways of financing health systems;

(2) estimate the order of magnitude of financial needs for the Strategy;

(3) promote, develop methodology for, and support cost-benefit and cost-effectiveness studies on health systems and technology;

(4) support developing countries on request in preparing proposals for external funding for health;

(5) use its mechanisms to identify needs and matching resources;

(6) coordinate the activities of the Health for All Resources Group, representing countries, intergovernmental, bilateral and multilateral agencies, and foundations, working together to rationalize the transfer of resources for health for all and mobilize additional funds if necessary.

20. WHO will pursue global programmes to foster and support the essential elements of primary health care in countries through the identification and generation of appropriate technology and the provision of guiding principles and training material for its delivery in the most efficient way through health infrastructures. Particular attention will be paid to areas of high priority for the implementation of the Strategy that have been neglected until now at the international level.

Global programmes for the essential elements of primary health care

21. Action at the *national level* will include:

Action at national, regional and global levels

(1) ensuring direct technical cooperation on request to support the implementation and evaluation of national strategies;

(2) ensuring the dissemination of relevant information to ministries of health and other relevant ministries and bodies;

(3) collaborating with the other United Nations agencies working in the country in support of national efforts for socioeconomic development as part of the national strategy.

22.   Action at the *regional level* will include:

(1) enlisting top-level political support in the region;

(2) regional coordination of the implementation, monitoring and evaluation of the regional strategy;

(3) promoting regional intersectoral action to support the strategy;

(4) ensuring the exchange of information among countries regarding the national and regional strategies;

(5) facilitating technical cooperation among countries;

(6) organizing technical cooperation between WHO and its Member States;

(7) supporting national efforts at research and development in connexion with their strategies and coordinating regional research and development efforts in connexion with the regional strategy;

(8) supporting training;

(9) identifying resource needs and possible external sources for supplying them.

23.   Action at the *global level* will include:

(1) promoting top-level global political support for the Strategy;

(2) global coordination of the development, implementation, monitoring and evaluation of the Strategy;

(3) enlisting international nongovernmental and voluntary organizations within the health and related sectors to carry out specific tasks for the implementation of the Strategy;

(4) global enlistment of the support of other sectors through United Nations agencies, and through other intergovernmental as well as nongovernmental and voluntary organizations;

(5) ensuring interregional cooperation;

(6) identification, generation and dissemination of valid information on health systems and technology;

(7) global promotion and coordination of research and development in relation to the Strategy;

(8) organization of global programmes to support the Strategy;

(9) generation of guiding principles on technical and managerial matters based on national experience as well as related training material;

(10) global coordination of the international transfer of resources for the Strategy.

24. WHO staff members in countries, in regional offices and at headquarters will give top priority to work required for the Strategy.

WHO secretariat

25. The Director-General of WHO, in accordance with his constitutional role as chief technical and administrative officer of the Organization, subject to the authority of the Executive Board, will ensure that the Secretariat at all operational levels provides the necessary support to countries, regional committees, the Executive Board and the Health Assembly for the implementation of national, regional and global strategies. The Director-General will also ensure that the Secretariat acts as an efficient instrument for giving effect to the resolutions and decisions of the regional committees, Board, and Health Assembly concerning strategies for health for all by the year 2000, and for carrying out those aspects of the national, regional and global strategies that are assigned to the Secretariat by these bodies.

The Director-General of WHO

IX. Conclusion

1.   The prospective socioeconomic and health background for the Strategy is a sober one. Yet the health and related socioeconomic policies to attain the goal of health for all by the year 2000 have been clearly defined. Ways have been described of giving effect to these policies at national and international levels by supporting the development of health systems based on primary health care and related multisectoral action. Illustrative targets have been identified. If the world's political, socioeconomic and health leaders are provided with suitable information, and heed this information, there is every reason to believe that the intercountry cooperation required to implement the Strategy will take place, and that the necessary resources can be generated and mobilized.

2.   The Strategy will not only contribute to health development throughout the world; it will contribute to and will derive strength from the International Development Strategy for the Third Development Decade and will thus help to establish the New International Economic Order. In spite of the seriousness of the problems involved and the complexity of the measures to resolve them, there is every reason for optimism that the Strategy can be implemented and that its successful implementation will be a landmark in the social history of mankind.

3.   To ensure implementation, debate has to give way to action. To this end, it is necessary to prepare a plan of action, including measures to be taken at country, regional, and global levels, not only within the health sector, but also within other sectors concerned. This serves to emphasize the importance of involving the United Nations Economic and Social Council and subsequently its General Assembly. These considerations led the Thirty-fourth World Health Assembly in May 1981, as the supreme organ of the World Health Organization representing all its Member States, to request the Executive Board of

WHO to prepare without delay a draft plan of action to implement the Strategy, for review by the regional committees of WHO at their 1981 sessions, finalization by the Board in January 1982, and submission to the Thirty-fifth World Health Assembly in May 1982.